NUTMEG AND MACE

MARIAN KIM

CONTENTS

MARIAN KIM

1

PROPERTIES

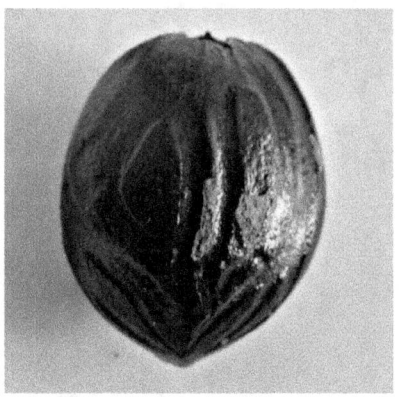

Nutmeg is made from the seed of the evergreen tree while mace is made from the covering of the seed.

Scientific name: Myristica fragrans

Other names: Magic, jatipatr and muscade

Nutrients: Vitamins A, B2 (riboflavin), B3 (niacin), B9 (folic acid) and C. They also contain minerals like calcium, copper, iron, magnesium, manganese, potassium and zinc.

Properties

Nutmeg and mace have:

Analgesic (pain relieving) properties

Antiseptic (antibacterial, antifungal) properties

Anti-depressant properties and carminative (anti-flatulent) properties

Nutmeg also has antioxidant properties which protect the cells from the free radical damage that causes premature aging and degenerative diseases.

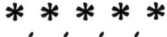

2

USES

Diarrhea treatment

Nutmeg and mace are used for diarrhea. Powdered nutmeg is mixed with honey to treat diarrhea.

Nausea treatment

Nutmeg decoction with honey is used to treat nausea and indigestion. A tea made from nutmeg, mace and slippery elm is mixed with cream, boiled and drunk when lukewarm to reduce nausea and indigestion.

Flatulence treatment

Nutmeg and mace are used for flatulence (intestinal gas). A tea made from nutmeg, mace and slippery elm is mixed with cream, boiled and drunk when lukewarm to ease flatulence. Nutmeg and mace are also used for abdominal pain.

Kidney disorder treatment

Nutmeg and mace are used for kidney disorders. Nutmeg is thought to be beneficial for removing kidney stones.

Insomnia treatment

Nutmeg and mace are used to treat insomnia (sleeplessness). Nutmeg powder is mixed with warm milk to aid in relaxation and sleep. Nutmeg powder can also be mixed with ghee and applied to the forehead to induce sleep.

Rheumatism treatment

Nutmeg and mace are used to treat aching joints and rheumatism since they have analgesic properties. Nutmeg oil can be used to massage the joints and relieve the pain. It is also used for sciatica and neuralgia (nerve pain).

Muscle ache treatment

Nutmeg oil can be used to massage aching muscles and relieve the pain.

Menstrual pain treatment

Nutmeg powder mixed with honey is consumed to reduce menstrual cramps. Nutmeg also stimulates menstrual flow.

Mouth sore treatment

Nutmeg and mace are used to treat mouth sores.

Toothache treatment and prevention

Nutmeg and mace are used to treat toothaches. Nutmeg has compounds which can kill tooth cavity forming bacterial in the mouth.

Halitosis treatment

Nutmeg and mace are used to treat halitosis or bad breath because of their antiseptic properties. Nutmeg or mace powder can be sprinkled on a toothbrush when brushing the teeth for their antibacterial effect.

Colon cancer prevention

Nutmeg and mace contain myristicin which is said to prevent the growth of colon cancer.

Alzheimer's disease prevention

Nutmeg contains myristicin which can hinder some of the enzymes that contribute to the development of Alzheimer's.

Acne treatment

Nutmeg powder is mixed with honey and milk powder to form a paste that is applied to the skin to treat acne. The milk powder can be replaced with orange lentil powder to from the acne paste.

Hemorrhoid treatment

Grated nutmeg is mixed with lard to make an ointment for hemorrhoids.

Asthma treatment

Mace powder is mixed with honey to treat asthma. Nutmeg oil is also inhaled to manage respiratory infections.

Depression treatment

Mace is used for depression.

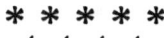

3

SAFETY PRECAUTIONS

1. Pregnant women should not use nutmeg and mace since they can cause miscarriages and birth defects.

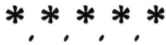

4

DRUG INTERACTIONS

1. Persons taking phenobarbital should not use/avoid nutmeg and mace since they can increase how quickly the body breaks it down and thus decrease its effectiveness.

2. Persons using medications which are broken down by the liver should not use/avoid nutmeg and mace since they can increase the speed at which the liver breaks down the medications. Examples of these medications include haloperidol (Haldol), imipramine (Tofranil), olanzapine (Zyprexa), propranolol (Inderal) and theophylline.

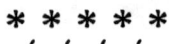

5

COOKING TIPS

Flavor: Warm spicy and sweet

Goes well with: Vegetables e.g. broccoli, Brussels sprouts, cauliflower, carrots, desserts e.g. pies and muffins with baked fruits, sausages, meat dishes, soups, stews

Tip: For best results buy whole nutmeg fruit and grind it yourself.

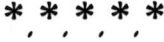

6

HERBAL RECIPES

Nutmeg Tea

Equipment

Tea pot or kettle

***

Ingredients

1 teaspoon of nutmeg and/or mace powder

1 cup of boiling water

Honey to taste (optional)

***

Instructions

1. Put the nutmeg and/or mace in a tea pot or kettle, add the boiling water and let it steep while covered for 10 -15 minutes.

2. Add honey (if using) to suit your taste before drinking.

*****

Nutmeg and Mace Decoction

Equipment

Non-reactive heavy saucepan

***

Ingredients

1 oz (30 grams) nutmeg and mace

1 pint (500 ml) water

***

Instructions

1. Place the nutmeg, mace and water in the saucepan, cover them and slowly bring the mixture to a simmering boil for 20 minutes.

2. Remove from the heat source and let the mixture cool to drinking temperature.

3. Strain the mixture, measure it and pour the liquid into a clean saucepan.

4. Heat the liquid until it begins to steam. Reduce the heat and let the liquid continue to steam until it is reduced to half its original volume. This may take 45 minutes to 1 hour.

5. Pour the decoction into a clean bottle.

6. Store the decoction in the refrigerator to lengthen its life.

*****

Nutmeg Tincture

Equipment

Glass jar with tight fitting lid

Dark tincture bottles

Cheesecloth

***

Ingredients

7 oz (200 gm) of nutmeg and/or mace powder

30 oz (1 liter) of 80-100 proof vodka

***

Instructions

1. Fill 1/3 of the glass jar with the nutmeg and/or mace.

2. Add the vodka to completely fill the jar to the top.

3. Seal the jar and label it with the date of preparation and name of spice used.

4. Store the glass jar in a dark place for 6 weeks ensuring that you shake them weekly.

5. After 6 weeks strain out the nutmeg and/or mace with a cheesecloth and pour the tincture into dark tincture bottles.

6. Label the tincture bottles with the date and name of spice used.

7. Store your herbal tinctures away from light and heat.

*****

Nutmeg Poultice

Equipment

Cheesecloth or old cotton sheet strips

***

Ingredients

1 tablespoon nutmeg powder

Boiling water

***

Instructions

1. Add enough boiling water to the nutmeg to wet it and make a thick paste.

2. Spoon the nutmeg paste onto the cheesecloth (or bed sheet strips) to make the poultice.

3. To use, apply the poultice to the affected area and cover with another piece of hot, wet cloth. Replace the hot, wet cloth when it cools with another hot one to keep the poultice hot.

*****

Nutmeg and Mace Infused Oil

Equipment

Double boiler

Large glass bowl

Sieve and cheesecloth

Sterilized dark jars

***

Ingredients

16 fl oz. (500 ml) vegetable oil like organic olive, sweet almond oil or sunflower oil

8 oz. (250 grams) nutmeg and mace

***

Instructions

1. Place the nutmeg, mace and oil in the glass bowl ensuring that the oil covers the spices. Simmer them in a double boiler for 1 hour at around 120 degrees F (49 degrees C). Do not let the mixture boil. You can repeat this step several times after letting the oils cool to create more concentrated herb infused oils.

2. Strain the mixture through the sieve and cheesecloth into a clean, dark jar ensuring you squeeze out as much oil as you can from the cheesecloth.

3. Label your jars and store your nutmeg and mace infused oils in the refrigerator and use them within 3 months.

*****

Nutmeg and Mace Salve

Equipment

Double boiler

Large glass bowl

Sterilized dark jars or tins

***

Ingredients

8 oz. (250 ml or 1 cup) nutmeg and mace infused vegetable oil (see previous recipe)

1 oz. (30 grams) beeswax

10 drops essential oils like lavender essential oil (optional natural fragrance)

***

Instructions

1. Place the beeswax, nutmeg and mace infused oil in the glass bowl and melt them in a double boiler.

2. Once melted remove from the heat source, allow to cool and add the essential oils (if using).

3. Pour the melted oils into the storage jars or tins and allow to cool completely.

4. Store the salves in a cool dark place.

***

Tips

1. Nutmeg and mace salve can be massaged onto aching joints and muscles.

###

ABOUT THE AUTHOR

Marian Kim is an experienced alternative medicine practitioner.

*****

OTHER BOOKS BY THE AUTHOR

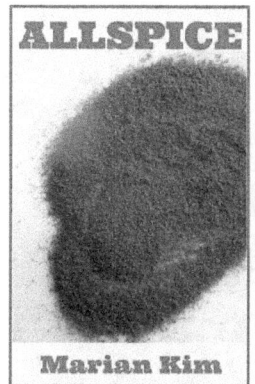

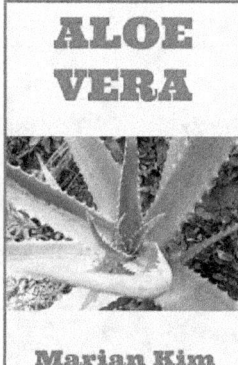

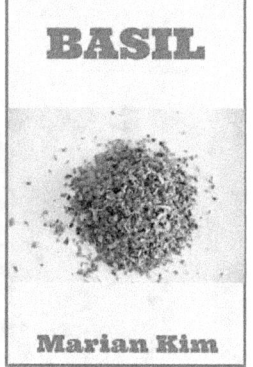

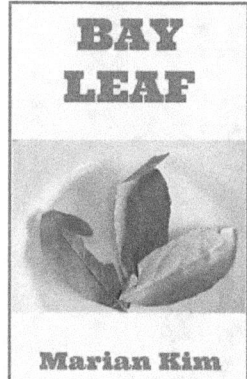

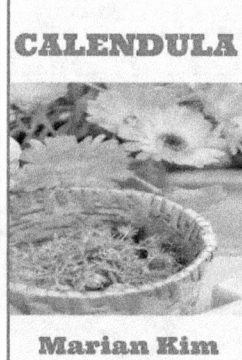

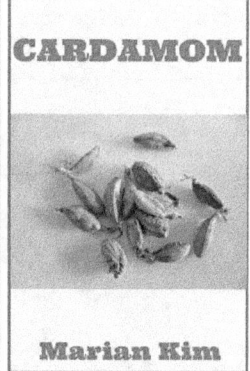

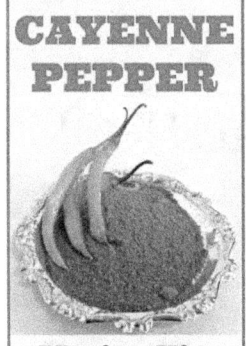
CAYENNE PEPPER
Marian Kim

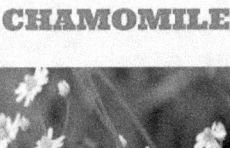
CHAMOMILE
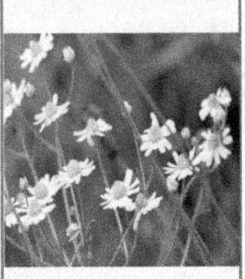
Marian Kim

CILANTRO & CORIANDER
Marian Kim

CINNAMON
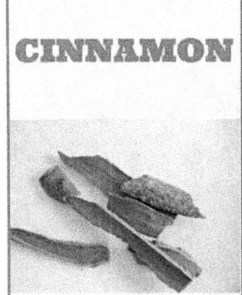
Marian Kim

CLOVES
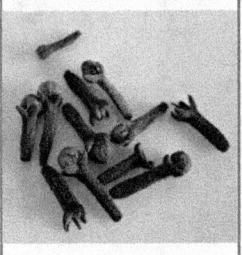
Marian Kim

CUMIN
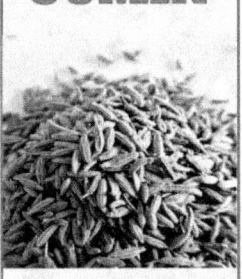
Marian Kim

DANDELION
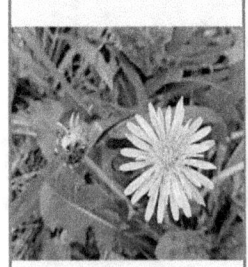
Marian Kim

DILL
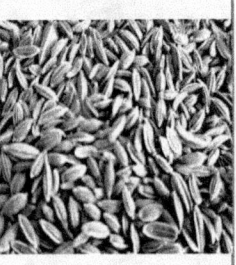
Marian Kim

ECHINACEA
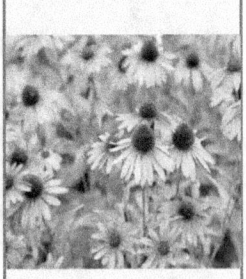
Marian Kim

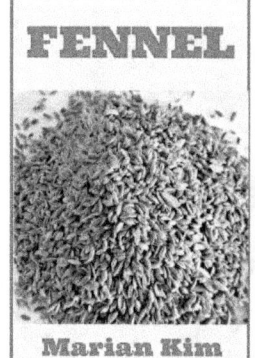

FENNEL

Marian Kim

FENUGREEK

Marian Kim

GARLIC

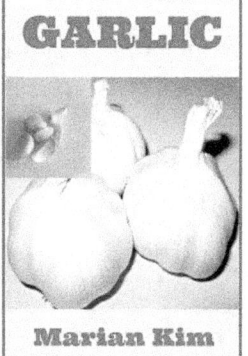

Marian Kim

GINGER

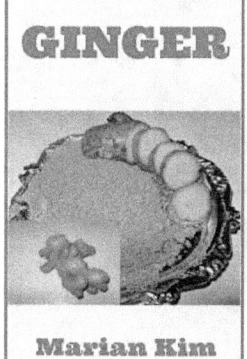

Marian Kim

GINKGO BILOBA

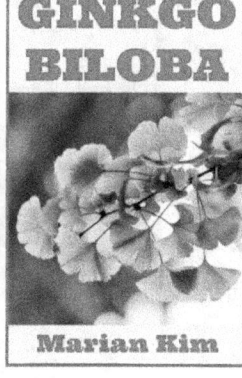

Marian Kim

GINSENG

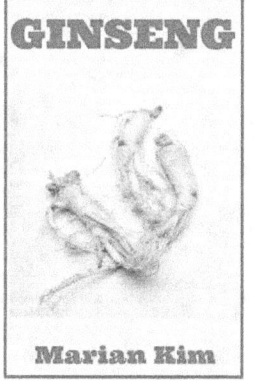

Marian Kim

LAVENDER

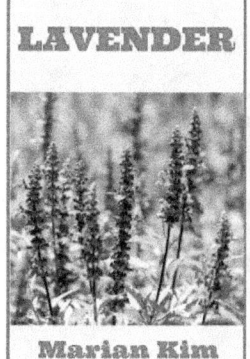

Marian Kim

MUSTARD

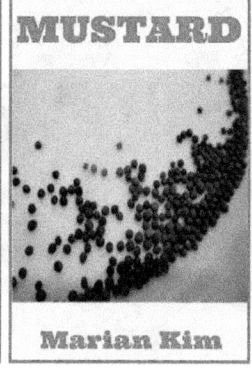

Marian Kim

NEEM

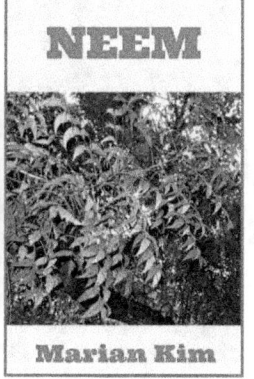

Marian Kim

NUTMEG & MACE

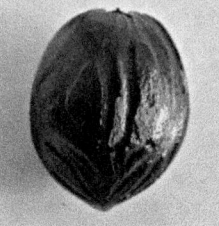

Marian Kim

OREGANO

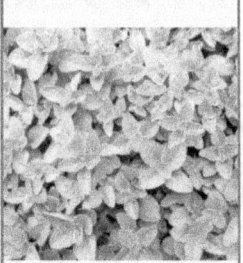

Marian Kim

PAPRIKA

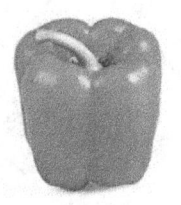

Marian Kim

PARSLEY

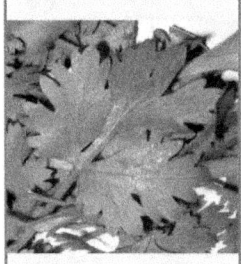

Marian Kim

BLACK & WHITE PEPPER

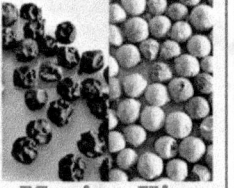

Marian Kim

PEPPERMINT

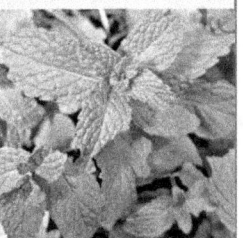

Marian Kim

ROSE HIPS

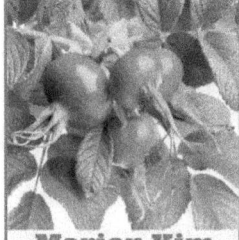

Marian Kim

ROSE PETALS

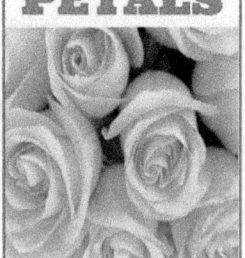

Marian Kim

ROSEMARY

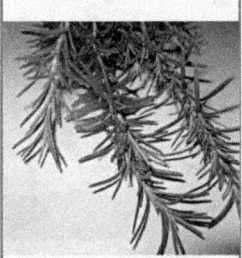

Marian Kim

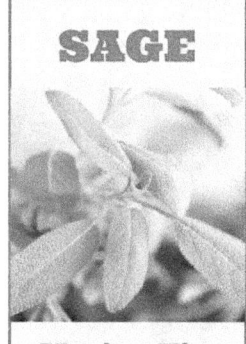

SAGE

Marian Kim

ST. JOHN'S WORT

Marian Kim

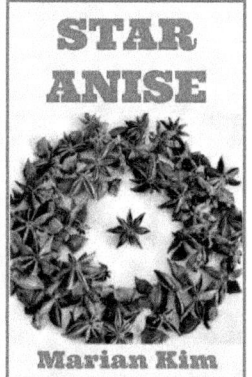

STAR ANISE

Marian Kim

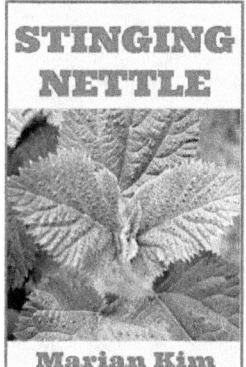

STINGING NETTLE

Marian Kim

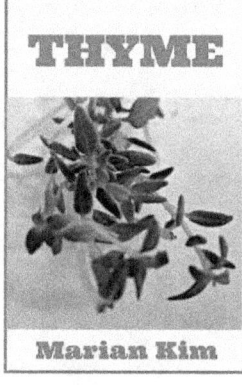

THYME

Marian Kim

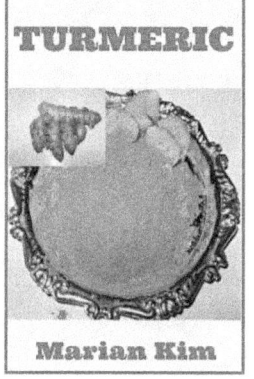

TURMERIC

Marian Kim

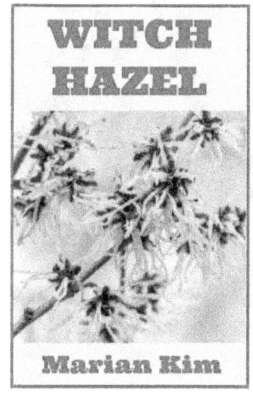

WITCH HAZEL

Marian Kim

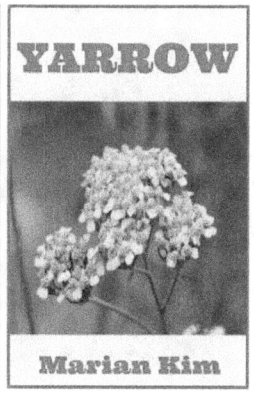

YARROW

Marian Kim

*****